Brain Bursts For All

Volume 2

A new concept, simple or profound

EILEEN FRY

THE CHOIR PRESS

First published in the United Kingdom in 2024 by

The Choir Press

ISBN 978-1-78963-514-0

Introduction

This book is to provide you with fun, pleasure and your own *Brain Burst*. It is for the creative mind. Study each story along with the illustration as a separate entity, pause for a while, then grab a pen.

If you are leading a group into creative writing or thought processing, it is up to you to go on a journey.

The group could be schoolchildren, or seniors needing guidance, or just on their own they could study it and find pleasure.

The book could be a useful gift to a loved one then you can share your own *Brain Bursts* together. If it makes you smile, then it is worthwhile.

Finally, I must remind you that however you use the book, the conclusions you reach are subject to your own interpretation.

Enjoy!

Love and blessings

Eileen Fry

Eileen Fry is an established author, but this book is a new concept. Her previous books have all been historical ghost stories and childhood autobiographies. She worked for many years with children with special needs and then most recently cared for her husband with Alzheimer's.

Dedication

This book is dedicated to Mike, my husband.

With thanks to everyone at St Oswalds Village especially Marshall and Michael

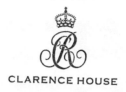

CLARENCE HOUSE

12th February, 2024

Dear Eileen,

So many thanks for your very kind letter and for your generous words of support and encouragement, which were greatly appreciated.

Thank you also for the copy of your book, "Brain Bursts For All", which I much look forward to reading.

With best wishes

Camilla

Poetry cafe
Gloucester
Library
01452 426973

Eileen's 'Brain Bursts' is the perfect coffee break read. I'm reading it sat in the library and wondering now about all the little moments of creative thought I have in a day that go unnoticed. I wonder what I would write about if I put pen to paper?

I really like "A Robin" who signals a "hello mum" to me. My favourite is "The silent witness" - the words of a tree giving out peace and protection to those taking shelter under it. Eileen's lovely musings have inspired me to pause for thought more, to notice the world around me ... and maybe even share those thoughts. I love Eileen's idea of using her bursts as conversation starters. What a lovely

: Martha. x

Dear Eileen,

Thank you very much indeed for your truly excellent leaflet. The words, the pictures and the ingenious links between them are genuinely inspirational.

It made me think deeply about our human thought processes: the way our brains actually work: spontaneous thought; generative thought; associational thought; inspirational thoughts and creative thought.

With our warmest wishes,

Lionel and Patricia

Lionel Fanthorpe
Cardiff Author T.V. Presenter etc.

Butterfly Love

My butterfly mind flits from place to place.

Bad thoughts, good thoughts most of all,
must-do thoughts.

Will it ever settle into calm?

The only time the butterfly settles on a soft
firm place of rest is when I think of you and
the love we share.

Calm restored.

Reason for living. Life's purpose revealed.

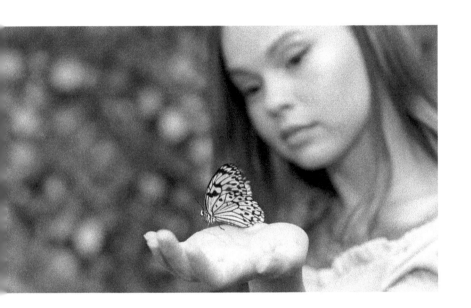

The Duvet

The duvet is a divine discovery

Snuggle, wriggle or just lie still

Succumb to its warm light cover

Tender bliss just encourages rest

Gentle, kind and all-embracing

Much nicer than even an eiderdown.

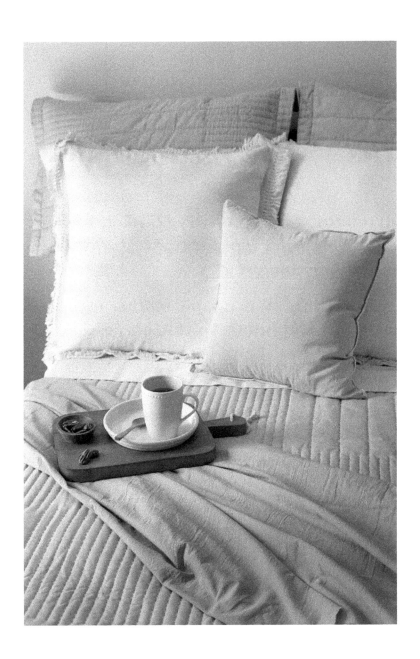

The Blanket

As a baby, I loved a furry blanket. I would clutch a corner, hold it tight. Stuff it in my mouth for comfort.

One balmy evening, my mother wanted to cure this bad habit. That night, a sheet was my only cover. I cried tears of angry frustration, until …

My cot was next to my parents' bed. My little baby arm pushed through the bars of my restrictive cot and fumbled until I managed to grab their furry blanket and ram it in my throat. Problem solved.

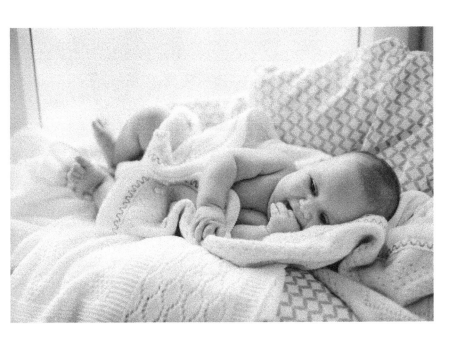

Glastonbury

Wall-to-wall music. Singing, shouting, laughing, crying. Crowd herding, all attempting to get close to the beats. Fighting off sleep in case of a miss. Stars named by their quirks, their eccentricities, praised, accepted. Fashions bright, colourful, anything goes. High heels, boots, socks, bare feet, whatever. Tiny tents, temporary homes, ready for anything, love and fun all around. Instant friends. Place of origin, who cares, brother? Weather, what weather? Torrential rain or blistering heat, bring it on. Suddenly all is over; everything surplus is dumped. Back to the real world.

Or was Glastonbury the real real world?

See you next year.

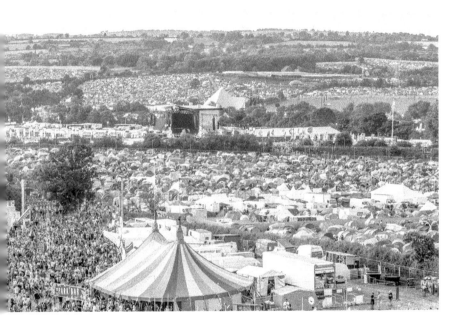

My Pretty Frock

That's a pretty frock!

Everyone admired it and said nice things about me.

Aunty Megan made the frock. It was knitted to perfection. Delicate pink stitches decorated with an angora fluffy cat.

I sat on a seat for a proper photographer.

I was so happy.

Time passed quickly.

My frock became small,

I now had to wear a dress.

It was sad when my frock became a dress. Was it because of the war?

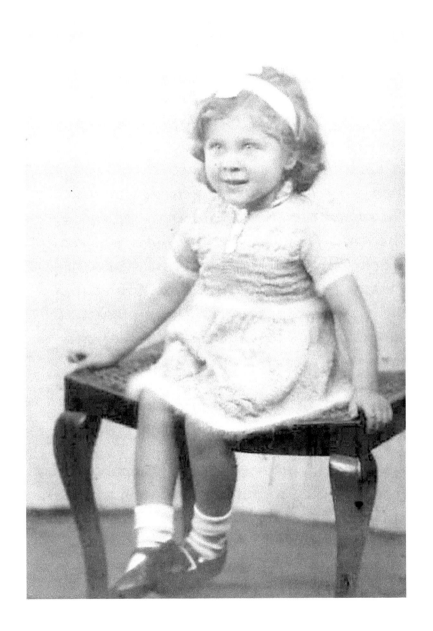

Saturday Nights

Saturday nights were special. The radio switched on, "In Town Tonight" was the first programme. There was always a fun story about London. Mum got out the tablecloth. The week's sweet ration was put into a bowl. The playing cards were out. This meant business. "Saturday Night Theatre". This was the late show, not really for children. Our Saturday night was when I was with my mum and dad. Sometimes, the plays were scary. They were meant, it seemed to me, to send you to bed afraid to close your eyes in the dark, for fear of a re-enactment. I refused to show any fear in case I missed out on next week's treats. I still wanted to be up for the challenge.

I well remember the play "Jamaica Inn". It seemed just so real. Years later, when on holiday, I persuaded the family to go there. I stepped inside the old remote den of iniquity with trepidation, but kept the fear I felt on both occasions to myself.

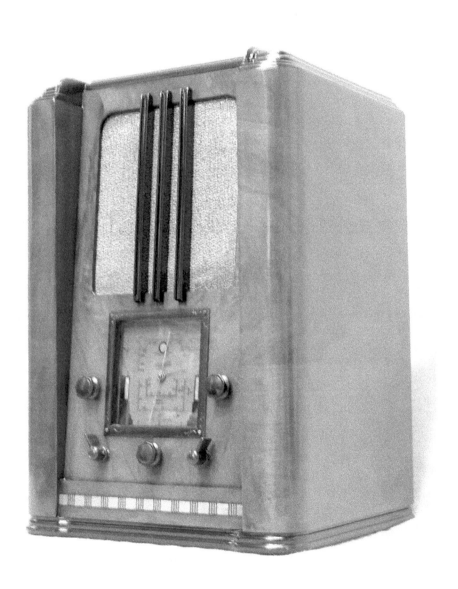

The School Playground

The girls together in a group were talking about boys. Joan started it with a single remark. 'Wish I was a boy!' Soon, a few others joined in.

'Yeah, it's not fair, boys can go out to play with a football after tea and girls have to stay indoors and help.'

Another voice piped up. 'And I don't see why I must keep myself clean and tidy, when my brother comes home with a dirty shirt and torn trousers, just because he has been having fun. My brother pinches me and pulls my hair, then I have to clean his shoes and his football boots too.'

'I have to take my baby brother for a walk in his pushchair,' said Betty. The girls agreed it was better to be a boy than a girl.

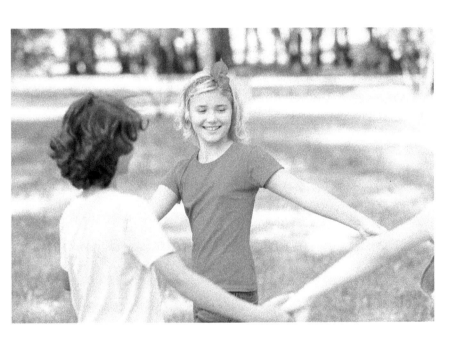

The Stepping Stone

On a pathway alongside the river. Lightly, she placed her sandalled foot on the stone, laughing on her way. Not a care in the world.

Under the stone, if anyone had cared to examine, was a little damp world of its own making.

Damp black soil was home to a myriad of ants, insects and creepy crawlies.

Whose secret world did you step on unwittingly as you made your journey of progress?

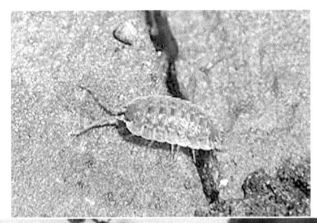

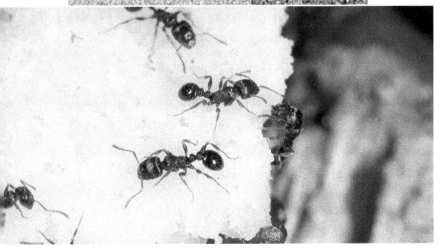

Too Busy for Love

I long for that special moment, that connection. Instant love across a crowded room, or maybe a silent library. Who knows? When and if it happens, will I be too busy to stop and recognise that moment when time stands still?

My worry is I will be too busy or too preoccupied.

Will I be texting or taking a call? Shall I be rushing to catch a bus or looking for a half-price bargain?

When that as yet unknown man speaks, shall I be gulping a coffee? Shall I say, 'Sorry, I have an appointment with the hairdresser'? Will I miss my chance?

Have I missed it already? Just let me recognise the moment.

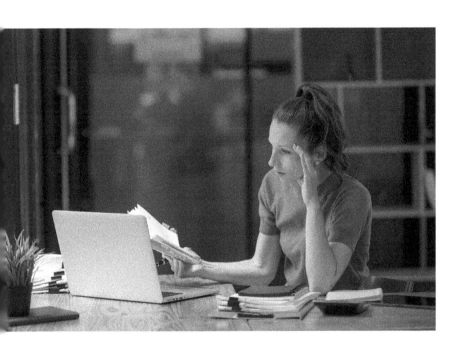

Ups and Downs

Crossing a mountain can be a very tough call, especially if you just expected a country walk.
Crossing a busy road in a big city, just as challenging.

Highs and lows, our lives can be similar.
We need a bit of thought and planning to get to the other side.

Make life your own special journey,
use the lows and embrace the highs.

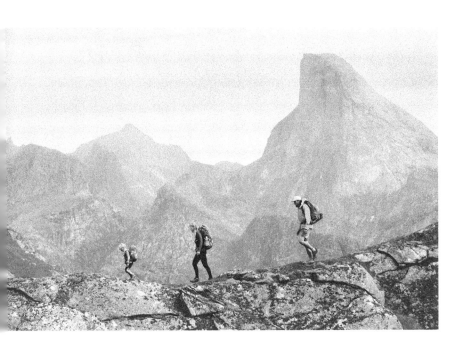

What is this thing called love?

Love has many aspects.
Sometimes beyond our own understanding.
Do we deserve love ever when we withhold
it?
Can we give love or even recognise it?
Love, of course, can be between two people.
Eyes meeting across a crowded room. The
dream!
Love can be a simple act of kindness.
Helping with the washing-up. Shopping for
someone unable to cope, especially when it's
raining.
Assisting a stranger in the supermarket,
reaching up to a top shelf beyond their
stretch. Just take care!
Love is giving a smile to a glum, grumpy,
unattractive bag of bones.
Love is patiently listening to a complaint
even if it is not your fault.
Love is offering to cut Granny's toenails.
Okay, but it's true.
Finally, love is saying thank you for all we
have in our own life.

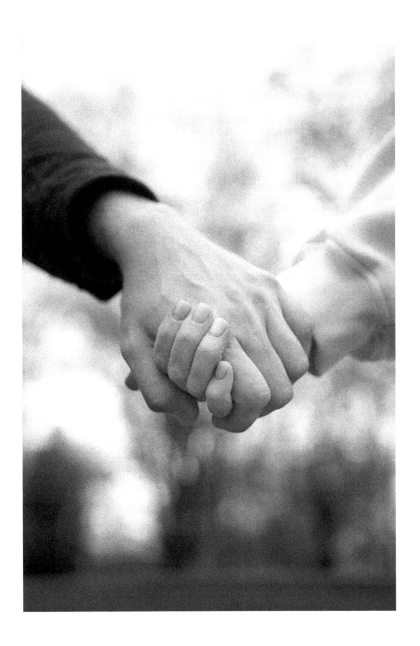

Your Smile is as False as my Teeth

Your smile is as false as my teeth
and your 'Have a nice day'
fools me none.
I know you are handsome,
and your eyes are divine,
but counting out numbers, the plus is all
mine.
I get the word 'scam',
and my nose smells a rat.
My money is hidden,
it's under my hat,
and your smile is as false as my teeth.

So 'You have a nice day,'
try your luck somewhere new.
When I'm leaving my money,
it won't be to you.

Get out of my life now,
and 'the pleasure's all mine'.
I can add up the numbers and I'm still
feeling fine.

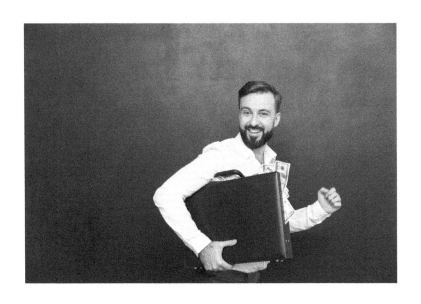

A Busy Bee

Making angry noises.

Trying to rush around

and make my presence felt.

Ignore my warning at your peril.

I will be noticed.

If you cross my path, I will sting you!

I will give you pain!

Slow as a snail.

The slimy snail is not so obvious.

He is no threat and is often ignored.

Look closely, his shell is beautifully made.

He perseveres and will get there in the end.

Do you know people like this?

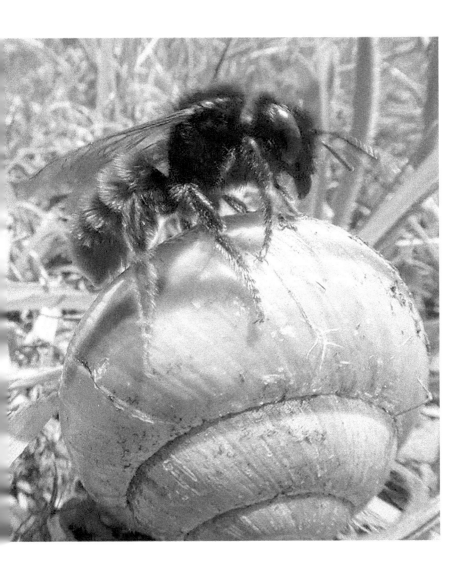

A Gargoyle, Ugly as Sin

Poor, poor sad face stuck forever in a
grimace.

What is his message, what is he thinking?

Pain and misery, or is he just scary?

Whatever his thoughts, they will not
change.

He is permanent but not pretty.

Did his creator want to bring us fear?

After posing, did he turn away and smile?

Is he just a fun creature playing a game?

When he was finished, did a workman just
put away his tools or smile and say,
'Goodnight, Fred. Now you are finished'?

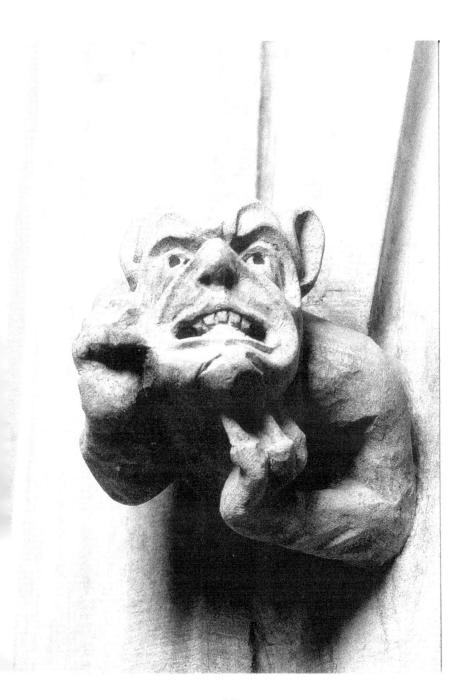

Alone Again, Naturally

Why am I alone?

Everyone else is having fun.
I have an assignment to do,
Words will not come.

I am very tired.

I am cold and alone.

I crash out on the sofa,
Wrap myself up, fall asleep.

I stagger to the kettle,
Make a cup of tea.

Then I find it.

A forgotten bar of chocolate.
Bliss!

Life has changed.

Chocolate has made a difference.
The world is great again.

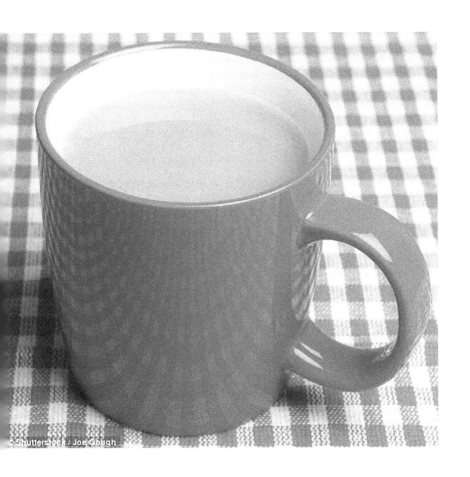

31

Spending a Night with Amy Winehouse

The pilot revved the engine,
Atlanta Airport fast becoming a distant
blur.
Two lone passengers now sitting together.
Smiled and settled. Heathrow was next.
In theory, they were a mismatched pair.
A middle-aged grandma leaving Dot in
Virginia.
The eye-stopping girl had elaborate, dark
piled-high hair.
Eyes made up, tattoos and a fab frock.
She had left New Orleans and a trail of
tumultuous tales behind her.

But in no time

Hushed but confidential and constant.
Conversations never to be shared were
taking place.
Creative pens began as their first common
bond.
The grandma promised to be Mum for the
night as they both slept.

Now Heathrow was their new place.

Separation inevitable, they hugged goodbye.

How do I know? Well, I was the grandma.

A newspaper a while later told me all.

Amy Winehouse. 'Of course!'
Caring, talented, vulnerable and exploited, also sadly addicted.
But ... full of love, and giving the talents she had to others.

This had been my fun companion.
One morning, not long after her tragic death, I turned on the radio.

'Our day will come.' It was Amy singing, and I knew it was for me.

I cried and said thank you.

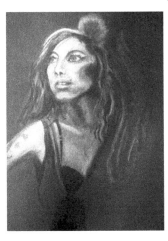

A New Baby

Last month, we were two. Now, we are three.
The world for us has changed.
Life now seen with new eyes.
A hungry little mouth that cannot wait is
ours.
The clock is gaining such speed.
We almost cried together last week.
Our little bundle looked up and smiled.
It was then we knew our reward.
This unique baby had chosen us.
May we be worthy of this special gift.

Oh dear, it's my turn to change the nappy.

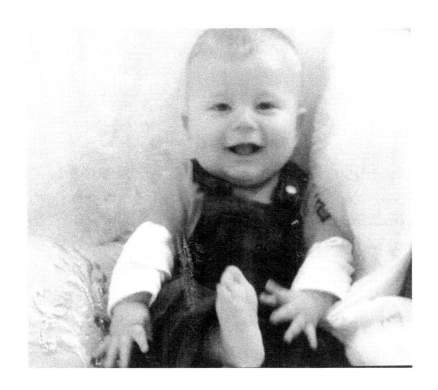

A Pen

Do make sure you have a pen at hand, and of course a scrap of paper. If not, you may miss a special connection with someone, or something essential. Random people, random tips, name of a book, or someone to do the best job at the best price. Okay, put it in your phone, but it's not the same as using a pen, even if it leaks in your pocket.

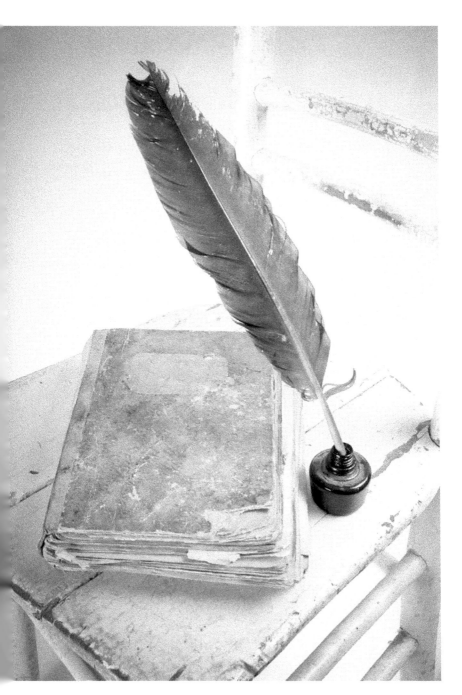

A Royal Wedding

Luke Bond and Robert Raikes

I settled down to see a royal wedding.
Half of Britain and USA eyes on the TV.
A wedding fairytale unfolded.

I heard a name I recognised.
It was Luke Bond the Windsor organist.
The same boy I once knew well.
A timid boy who tugged my arm.
Asking politely but firmly,
'Please can I play Robert Raikes?'

I had written a school play for junior
leavers,
Robert Raikes the name in history.
A Gloucester newspaper owner.
A family man who loved children.
He employed Mrs Critchley for a shilling,
to teach children to read on a
Sunday, their only day off.
Ninety children turned up in her cottage.
Teach them to read, what an idea!
Sunday school led to education for all.

Luke Bond was an excellent Robert Raikes.

The Royal Couple,
Meghan and Harry.
Luke Bond the organist and
Robert Raikes all came together.

What a surprise! What a connection!

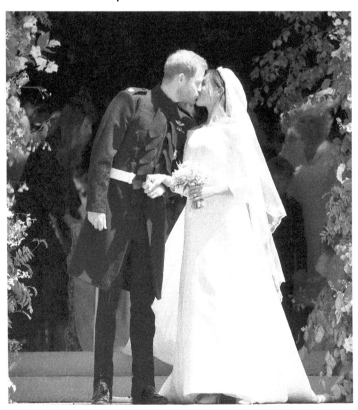

Bedtime

It's time to go to bed,

but there is always something else to do.

I just need a little more time. Even though I know I need to stop.

Okay, I give in, turn off the light and settle down.

Only to hear the ping of yet another message. Ugh!

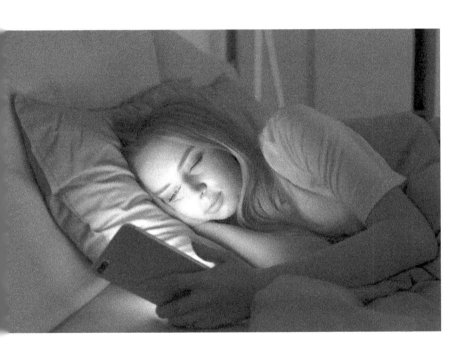

Clarification

I want it now.

I need answers.

Where? When? Why? How?

The mystery of life is a fog.

Long-lasting.

When I least expect it, the

sun bursts through.

Strong, bright and beautiful,

but I know I cannot

control those special moments.

I must seize answers when

they appear through the

haze of life

and be thankful.

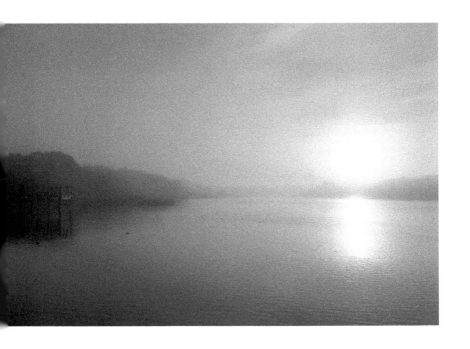

Egg on my Face

The chicken crowed loudly
as it laid the brown egg.

That was her job for the day.
She felt relief as it was taken.
Now it joined the many others.
The fresh brown egg was now
one of the many on their
way to a table.

Would it be used by a chef
to make a lemon sponge? Maybe.

Would it be dropped into
a pretty egg cup, only to
have its top smashed in,
consumed together with a
brown bread and butter
soldier dip? Delicious.

My egg appeared on my plate.
The vinegar made it quite special.
A pickled egg, washed down
with half a pint.

Now that is a treat!

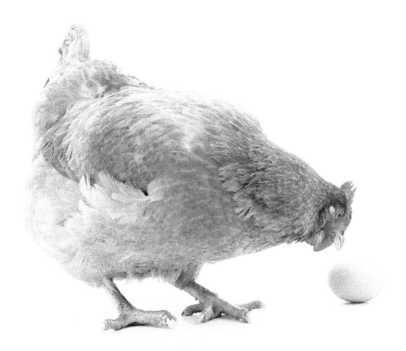

Fabius Pictor and False News

Fabius was a chronicler in ancient Rome. He wrote for his livelihood. It could be compared to News of the Day. Many of his tales are now buried into oblivion. Fabius used his pen sometimes to adjust facts. It has been suggested that the story of Romulus and Remus is questionable!

Some things never change.

Have you read a newspaper lately?

Think of Fabius Pictor and be cautious.

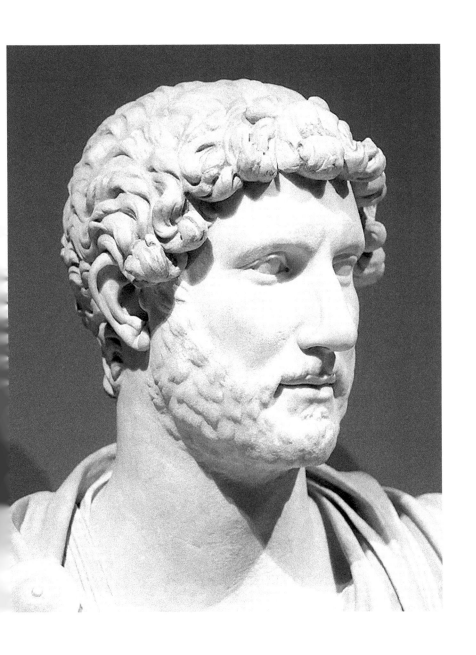

Father's Day

Captured forever.

Baby Jack and Daddy Paul.

A Father's Day photo.

What can be seen in their eyes?

Jack looks apprehensive.

His eyes say, Will I be able to cope?

Shall I understand, will I know my place?

Daddy Paul appears to be confident.

Quietly confident, passive acceptance.

His eyes say, Don't worry, son. I will help

you take it on.

As a father loves his son,

I am here for you.

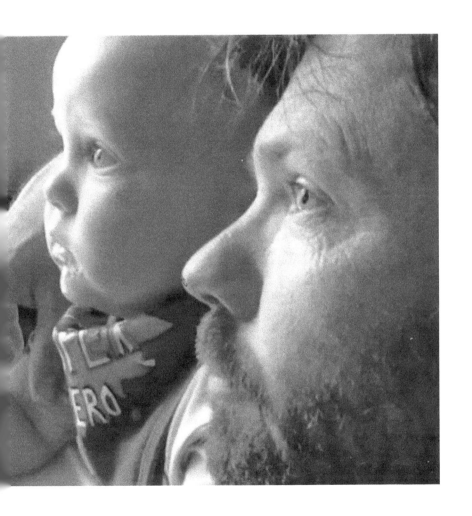

A Fishy Business

This was a tribute to a well-loved pet of twenty years.

The owner was heartbroken and could not find words.

On his behalf, his son Charlie Kyre almost became a poet.

The memorial stone was carved and erected.

Words written tell a poignant tale.

The emotional bond must have been important.

Perhaps the lucky old trout had a tickle just before a feed, a kindly few words.

This was Blockley in 1865.

Surely the only headstone ever for an old trout.

Well done, Charlie, you made an old man very happy.

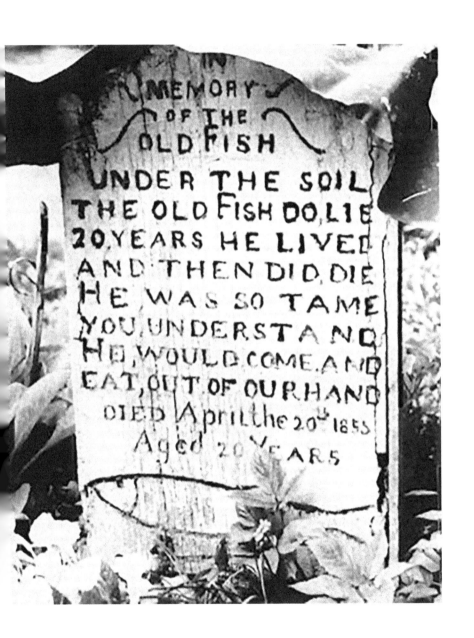

Holiday Spirit in Hot Sun

HOT SUN.
Hungry seagulls.
Happy surfers.
Hippies sweating.
Hopefuls singing.
Horizon shining.
Husbands smiling.
Hounds slinking.
Horses surfacing.
Humans sulking.
Hateful shouting.
Horrible smoking.
Hurting sunburn.
Hunky swimmers.
Heaving shops.
Hissing sandals.
Horrendous swimsuits.
Hop in the car.
Hometime.
Hurray!

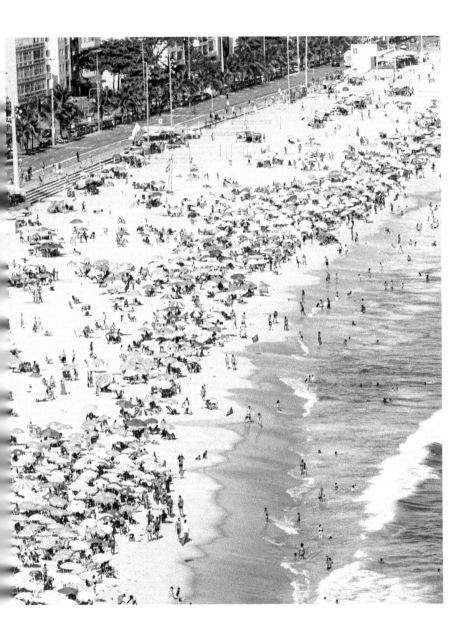

INDIAN CREEK, Kilmarnock, USA

Through the window I see a wonderful bay, luxury homes, superboats, but in my mind's eye coming into view is a canoe paddling along, inside, a native Indian.

Grey geese wildly passing by.

I can hear the threat of adventurous Englishmen searching for their own space.

They too seek a place to settle, but the same sunshine's warm rays, the same sky blowing clouds.

How can I ever focus on the truth?
INDIAN CREEK.

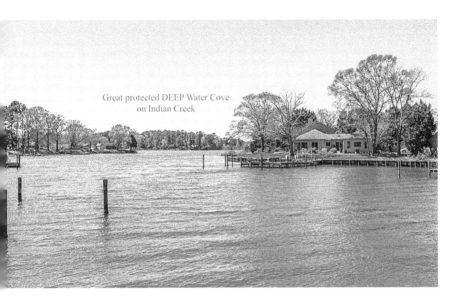

Great protected DEEP Water Cove
on Indian Creek

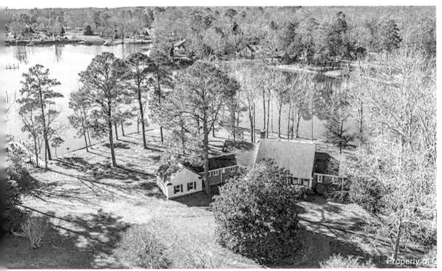

Property of C

Eugène Burnand
1850-1921

Le Paysan

I gazed at the picture of Le Paysan. The whole scene was now real. I was in that time and space, in that lane I stepped aside Chloe. Yes, Chloe the cow fixed her eyes on me.

We connected.

Jean-Claude the cowman did not notice me at all. Of course, I was invisible, but not to Chloe. No one will ever know our thoughts at that moment. The early sun was still, watery, and the day fresh and cool.

It was serene and blissful.

Then I was back in the real world.

Merci bien.

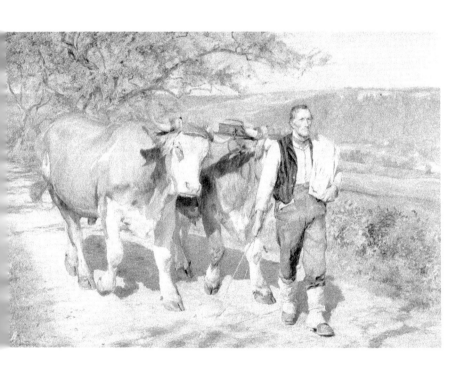

Make-Up

I love to use my make-up.

I can change my expression.

My eyes become larger.

Do I look more interesting now?
My alter ego comes to the fore,
my eyebrows a perfect shape.
This is the latest look.

I am bold, my lips larger.

My hair, of course, takes longer.
Brush, shape with a comb.

Volume and colour is vital.

Shall I add my clips? What a decision!
Eventually, my look complete.
My friend is waiting.

We are off to fairyland.

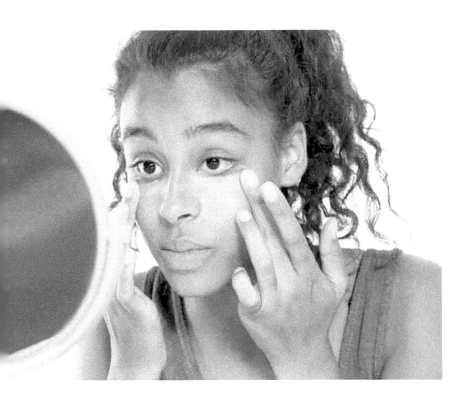

My Cat

I love my cat

I just love to stroke her
Sometimes she purrs so loud
Like a train at the station

Her face is adorable

Black with just a small patch of white
Green eyes with a mystical stare
I'm sure she sometimes smiles
She will happily on my lap

then quickly as she came

she is off, away to her world

not mine to know or share

When we are together, it is special

What's her name?

Tina

Don't ask me why

Oh drat, now she needs feeding.

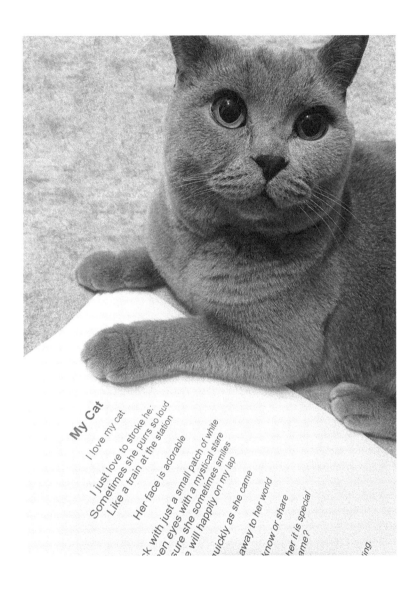

My First Love

The catch on the cot gave way to fumbling
three-year-old fingers. Now little chubby legs
made their way down the garden path.

The first adventure life had presented. A time for
decision. Through the garden gate, now down
the alley, across the path and over the road.

Opposite alley. Yes, this was right. Turn the
corner to delight.
This was the right place, rambling roses, grass
up to my knees.
He was there, playing quietly. I rushed in and
found such happiness.
I know we played with large deep pink rose
leaves. Making perfume. Absorbed, I followed
his instructions, crushing them into the enamel
pot.
Water now added, he offered the potion for me
to smell.
What bliss! It had all been worth the danger.
New freedom. The cup was heady.
I gazed into his dark brown eyes and felt my
first experience of love.

Shouting broke into the idyllic bliss of the
afternoon.
It was my mother, so pleased to find me. I had
never strayed before.
'She just wanted someone to play with,' his
mother said.
Even then, I knew it was more. Something
different.

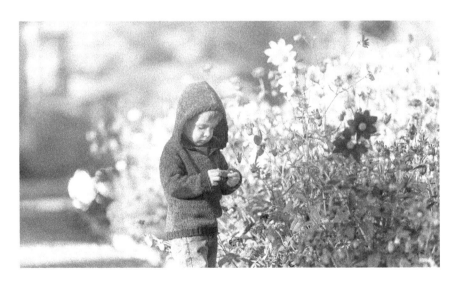

My Kingdom for a Horse

Cheltenham races a legend, an occasion
with no equal.
Initiation with the jet set.
Arabella decided to go for it.
Mad March had arrived.
Shopping for an outfit was a wow.
What a hat, no other like it!
Shoes amazing, with great heels.
Hairstyle trimmed, coloured and teased,
by Simon Perry himself.
Expensive, of course, but dreamy.
Arabella almost forgot to book a make-up
session,
but a window was tweaked in.
The day arrived. She was a vision in green.
Something to do with St Patrick.
Arabella felt lucky.

Then the blue clouds became black.
The heavens opened. She squelched back to
the far-off car.

Ah well, better luck next year!

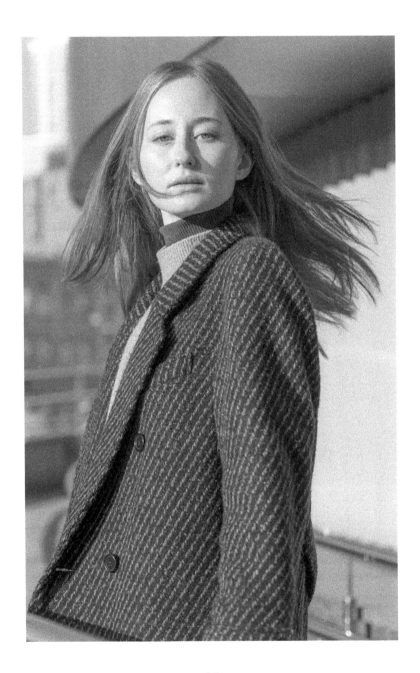

My Music

I love my music.

It helps me concentrate.

My mum doesn't understand.

To her, it is a loud racket.

I move with the beat.

I smile at the words.

My body jerks in tune.

Drums, keyboard, saxophone

hypnotise me.

Is that a shout to turn it down?

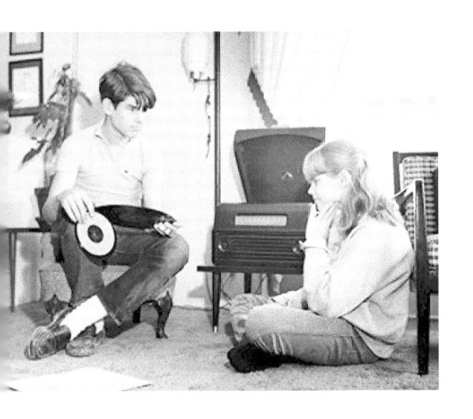

Never Give Up

Sometimes, even a small task seems impossible. I take a small step in what seems the right direction, but no, every path leads to nowhere. Then just as I decide to give up, I get a phone call. A friend suggests a different route. Why didn't I think of that? The truth is, we can do nothing on our own. So step back, let it go, start again, listen to that inner voice.

There is always HOPE.

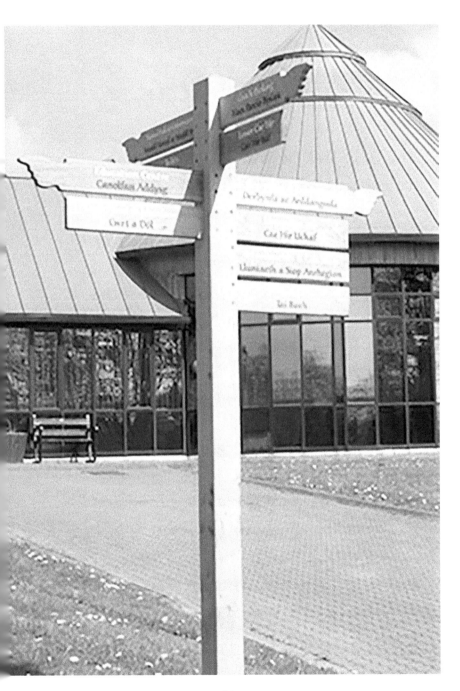

North Star

The first GWR broad gauge locomotive
Now standing still, his working days gone.

Sweat, blood and tears before he was
complete.
Ready to go, ready to blow, travel the
tracks.
If it could speak, it could recall fast
journeys.
The men who saw him take his first trip
were proud.
My grandad sweated and stoked factory
fires.
His eyes were droopy, large, bloodshot
As the years of labour progressed, but

I never heard him complain or wish for
A different life. Trains were in his blood.

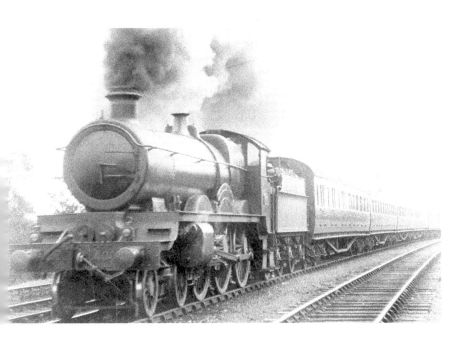

Only Good Tenants Allowed

There is a space to let in your head. It is fine to ask someone to step inside and look around. They may enjoy the visit, feel comfortable, but need more time to have a friendly discussion. If you allow them to become a tenant, will you profit from the experience? You must consider that what you treasure may become muddy and dusty, as they have different values. Don't let them into your space unless they appreciate your own interior choices. The wrong tenant may prove to give you grief and need to be evicted. Be strong when you decide.

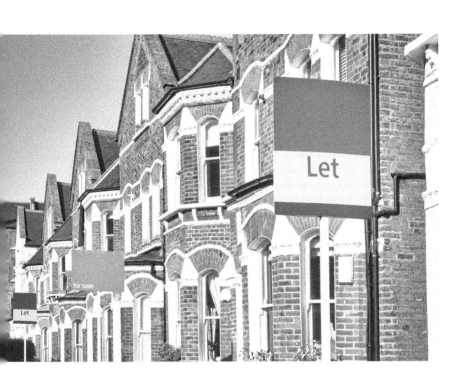

Piccadilly Circus

Back in the Day

Busy busy ever-busy Piccadilly.

Yesterday, today and tomorrow.

Somehow stopping, standing still.

A man, Frederick, stopped his van,

climbed out with a camera.

His job delivering clean laundry

in London stopped for a while.

He needed to capture a moment in time.

1947, just after the war.

What prompted him? I did not ask.

I just enjoyed the scene.

Frederick Cottrell was my father.

Thanks, Dad, for that day.

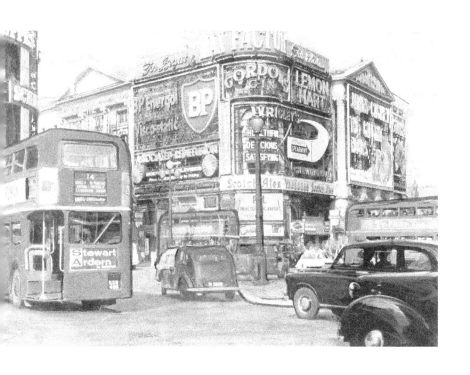

Prague

Prague is a beautiful city full of sights and sounds. Unforgettable buildings, monuments, bridges and steps. Cosmopolitan people, strange tongues, delicious food, quirky restaurants, relentless history.

On the other hand, there are some people who just book a flight to have their teeth fixed.

It takes all sorts to make a world.

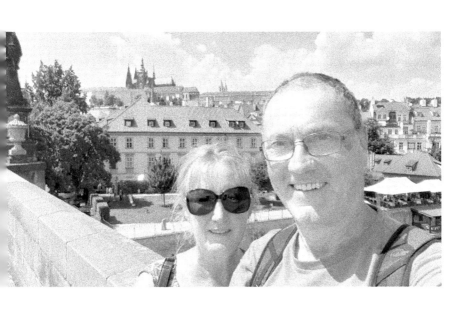

Put it in the Box

Time is a very strange thing. Past, present and future.

The past is how we see it.

On a good day, we look back with a grateful smile.

If it's a bad day, we feel sullen and angry and ask, 'Why me?'

However we view it, we cannot change our past, but how we deal with it can mould our future.

Put the past in a box lest it spoils your future.

Open a new box.

Live for today and enjoy it, not for what yesterday has taken away.

Hope for the future can give us so much joy, but just today can be a blast.

Smile, open up.

Giving love means you have a good chance of it coming back to you.

Go on, give it a try.

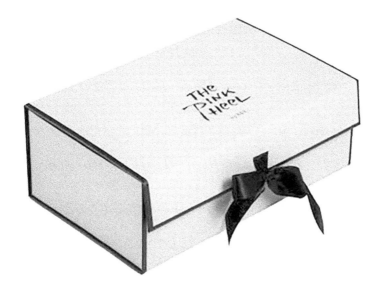

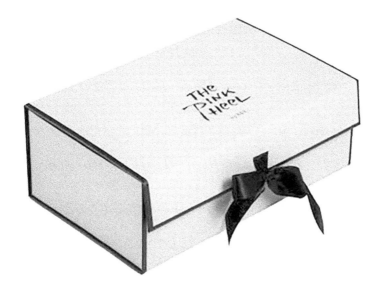

Resolutions

January is here. I must not delay
New Year resolutions must get underway

I tried it last year but it did not last long
So this time I intend to wise up, be strong.

I will try to be calm and not shout at all,
for instance, when muddy feet tramp in the
hall.

'Your slippers are there, dear. Do put them
on.'
I smile so sweetly then burst into song.

They think I have flipped, say it must be my
age
I think they prefer it when I am in a rage.

Know where they stand. Look and end with a
grin
Then put on their slippers, say it is not a sin.

I will send all the letters I owe and should
write
My fingers are cramped and I've been up all
night.

The postman is coming, papers slip through the door
One letter but nearly all bills on the floor.

I chat to a neighbour, the one who is odd

She probably thinks, You silly old thing.

But we have to keep trying. Make the world go around

Help others on Life's journey, that's what I have found.

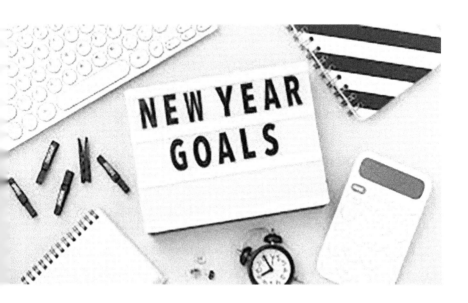

Tea at the Ritz

The photo tells all. A family enjoying tea at the Ritz.
They look perfectly at ease, suggesting that they do this often.
Later, the older lady poses with two gentlemen at hand.
What a performance! What a great day!

It was a first-time birthday surprise.
She had been whisked away one morning.
The drive involved a motorway, then a tube train to Knightsbridge.
Now up the magic steps to fairyland.
The fantasy world. The Ritz Hotel.
All things good or bad have to end.
Driven back home, still reeling with disbelief.
The birthday girl returned to her dear husband, who because of his Alzheimer's disease had been unable to join her.

I know because the old lady was me. I shall never forget that day.

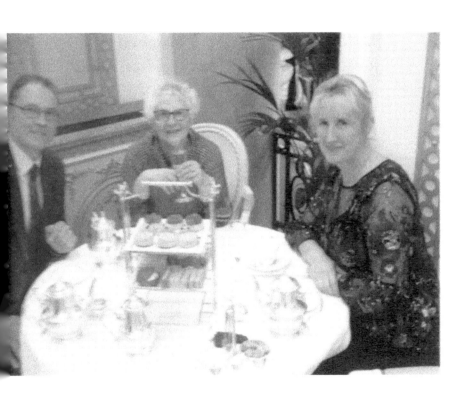

THE CHALLENGE

He spoke	She replied
challenged	blushed
questioned	checked her nails
paused	stared into space
trembled	cringed
stopped	crumpled
fidgeted	whispered
continued	pleaded
attacked	submitted
questioned	answered
justified	blinked
grimaced	remained calm
sweated	twisted
sat down	sat down

So there it was. She would get no rise.

She left, never to return.
He never found anyone suitable to replace her.

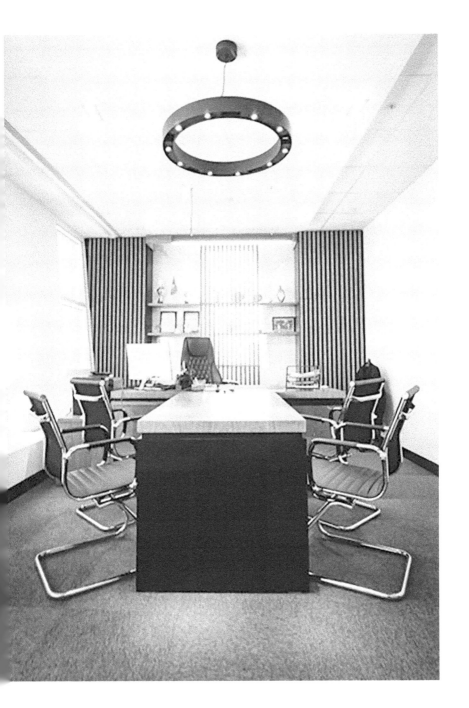

The Kettle

It reached boiling point
then just got hotter and hotter,
until it was no use to anyone.
Much as I had loved my kettle, it had to go.
I replaced it with a new model.

Now I am happy again.
Look out if you are always on the boil.
You may become redundant.

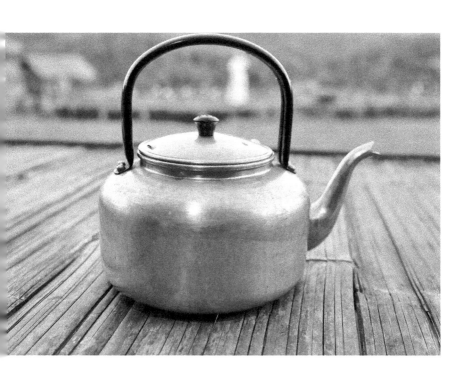

The Magnifying Glass

I had a bright magnifying glass

It was large and helpful

I was able to see again

My wisdom grew as never before.

Now help was at hand.

Time passed

My eyes became very cloudy

Even my precious glass did not help.

But I can still read between the lines.

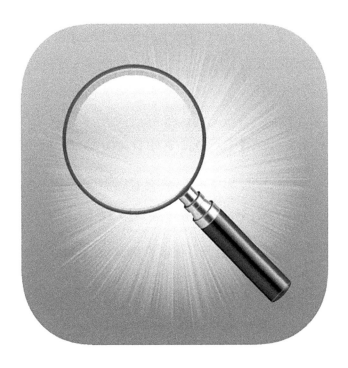

The Perfect Shape

I looked in the mirror. Oh dear.

I am not the perfect shape.

My bum is too big.

I need to lose an inch or two.

I walk into college hoping

no one is looking at me.

Molly is, dare I say it, fat.

We walked in together.

No one laughed at us.

So perhaps it is okay after all.

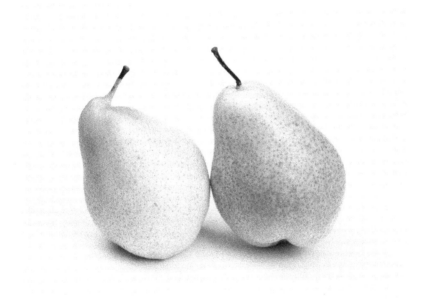

The Surgery before COVID

We sat in the surgery waiting for Doctor to be free,
No one said a word. It was quiet as could be.
I looked across the room, my face a blank look.
The person beside me was reading a book.
What a right miserable lot, I thought as I sat.
Just look at that woman, my word, she is fat.
That man has a cough and maybe the flu.
When will my turn come? I have so much to do.
The silence grew louder and I started to wriggle.
My tummy, it rumbled, and I wanted to giggle.
They all turned to me with glares horrified.
I was so embarrassed I felt I should have died.
Soon people were talking to hide up my shame.
I had not eaten breakfast. That must be the blame.
If you make an appointment to visit Doctor one day, Take heed of my warning is all I can say.

Nowadays, an experience like this is impossible due to progress.

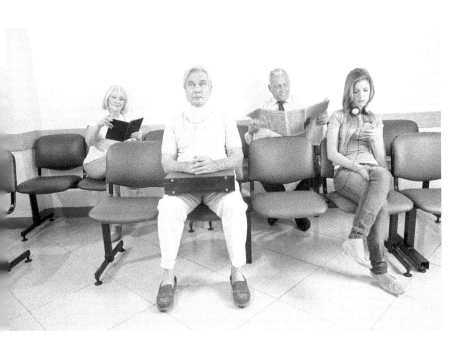

The Tape Measure

The blatant truth about a
tape measure is, it does not lie.
It wraps around my waist
as a silent critic.
I cannot even argue with it.
The reading is there for me
to deal with.
Shall I ignore the message,
pretend I do not care?
Or shall I now feel obliged
to take action?
I could look up all advice
out there on diets, healthy eating,
etc., all that is available.
Keep the results a secret
Decide nothing to be done
Or
Tell everyone I meet about
my problem.
Seek professional advice.

To lose or not to lose.
That is the question.

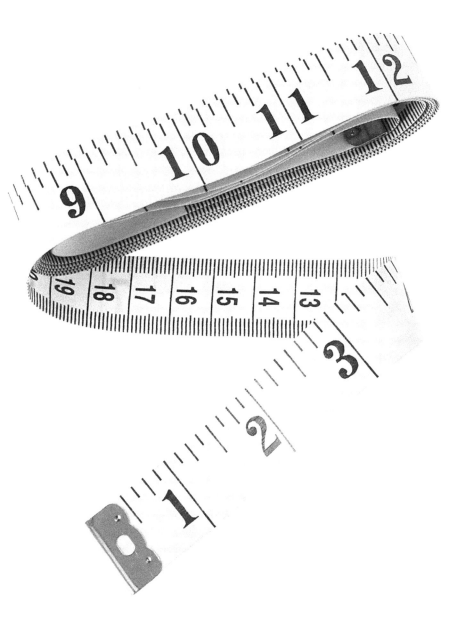

Today is your own Special Moment

Today, the weather will be right. Hot, cold, dry, or wet and windy. It will have its own beauty. Whatever happens today, we cannot choose the weather, only choose to embrace it.

When it's wet, we take an umbrella.

Wind needs to be confronted; it can be fun.

Snow has its own magic.

Sun can be strong and burn us if we don't protect ourselves.

Whatever the day has to offer, it will never come again.

So smile and enjoy.

Today is your special moment in time.

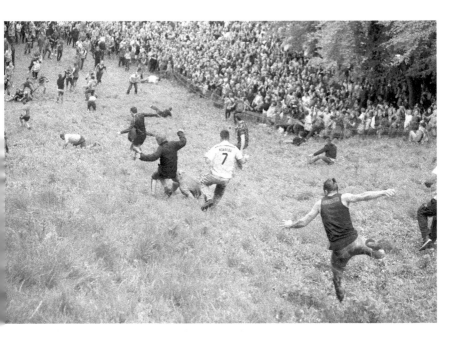

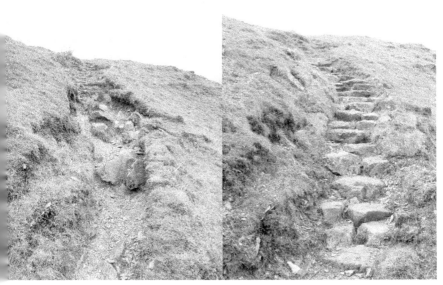

Truly an Amazing Bore

Christine loved the wonder of nature. She yearned to be part of it. A spring tide controlled by a lunar cycle sounded like something to be part of. A chilled March day in 2024 promised to be a five star. Bore on the River Severn in Gloucestershire. Camper vans travelled from far and wide, full of surfboards and all the gear. Fantastic! Christine put on her wetsuit to soar with a bore. As the time approached, she made her way but had to rush back for her paddle. Ten minutes later, all set, she returned to a nasty shock. The bore had been great but ten minutes early. Christine went purple with shock. Time and tide waits for no man, or woman either, it seems.

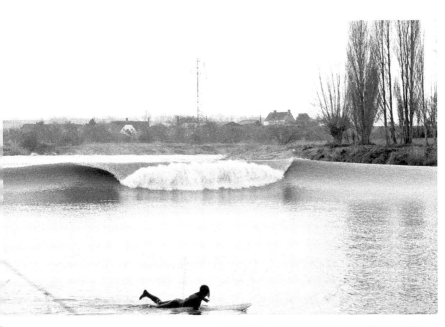

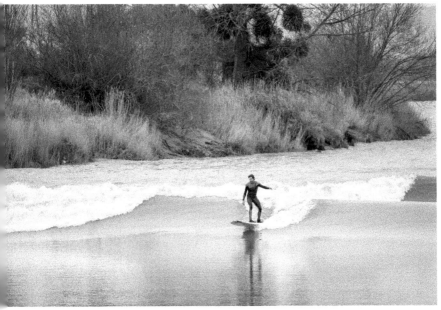

99

Walking on the Lines

I'm on my way,

I walk it every day

On my way to school, that is.

But this is the pavement,

The pavement with lines.

I know it's silly, so don't tell a soul.

I must not stop on the lines

Or my day will go wrong.

Don't laugh, it's tried and tested.

There! I've done it again.

Today will be a good one.

You see.

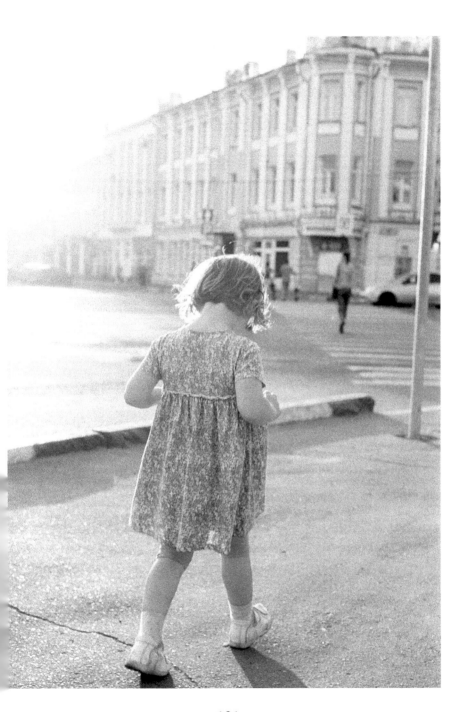

Back in the Day
Weston, Wonderful
Weston

A great adventure for the West Country.

Trip week and Swindon steam.

First week in July, mass exodus.

Trains shunting, engines blowing,
carriages heaving,
Beach full, deckchairs facing the sea.

Tide always out, fish and chips on good days.
Sandwiches, flasks of tea, ice cream if lucky.
Men with braces, trousers rolled up, no ties.
Children with busy buckets, castles
appearing.
Donkeys plodding up and down. Mum's
happy,
'Undressing' under a towel that is too small.
Laughter, noise, knotted hankies on hot
heads.
Now that is something to remember.

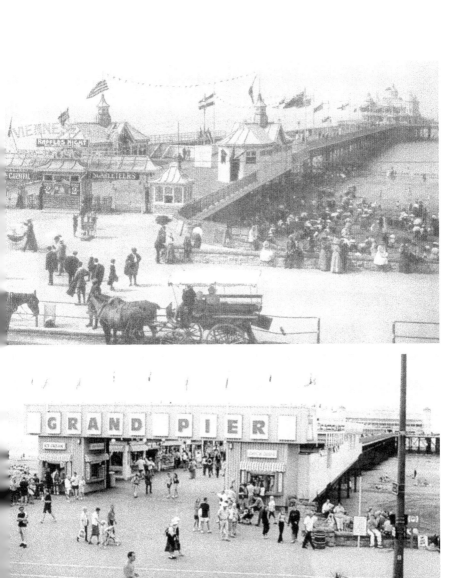

What Next?

I am a confused cat on an adventure.

My owner, Dick, vowed to take me.

We have walked a journey

Not alone but walking, walking.

Then on a boat, "Old Father Thames",

Someone shouted.

Now bells are ringing.

'Maybe the Bells of St Clement's,' said Dick.

'We shall soon be there.'

I purr as Dick keeps me warm.

What next? I wonder.

I often ask myself the same question.

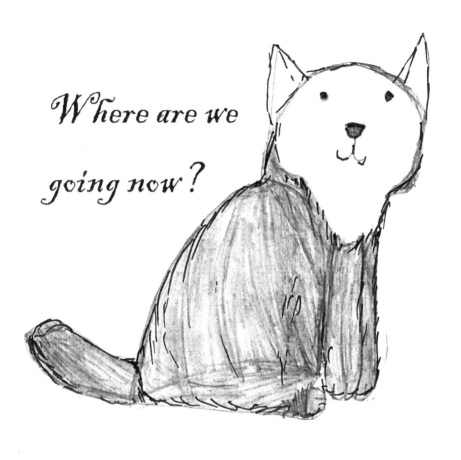

Where are we going now?

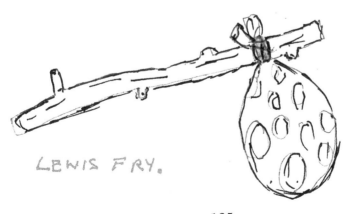

LEWIS FRY.

Something

Something tells me there's a trunk road ahead.

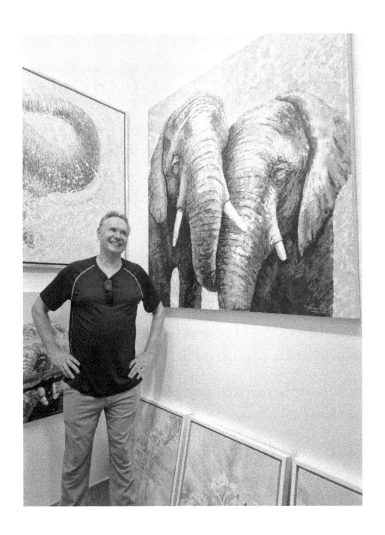

Harmony in Colour

Two large lovable dogs, one black, one white, but united. Musical notes, one black, one white, played together; the sound magical.

Reading a newspaper, white paper, black words printed.

Two colours needing each other, making us understand, see clearly.

Black people, white people, working together.

Result, amazing.

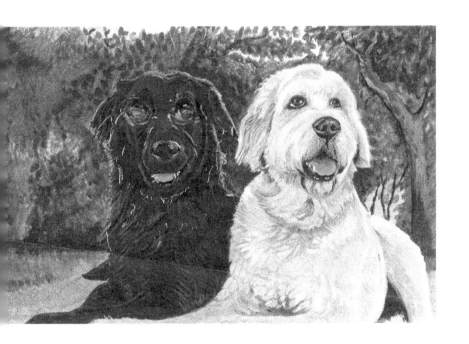

Mother's Day 2024

I woke up sleepily, went to the kitchen feeling the need for a cup of tea. I saw an already opened card and remembered it was Mother's Day. "Polly put the kettle on, Sukey take it off" again played in my head as the kettle boiled. Unexpectedly, I was then a small child sleeping in a musty shelter. My mother made the sign of the cross on my forehead with her damp light finger. She lay almost on top of me for protection as a night raid rumbled above. Now I know whatever happened or will take place in the future, I am a child of GOD.

Thank you, Mum x

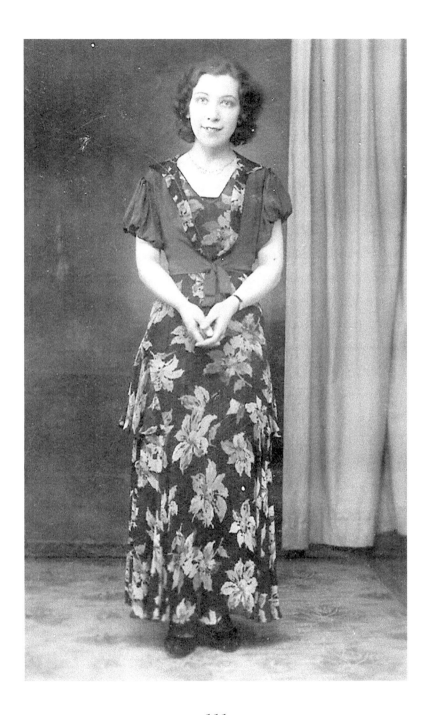

111

£10,000
The Winner

The 28th of November 1989 began as just an ordinary day. Anne was coming round with baby Hannah for coffee.

The phone rang as we sipped coffee and passed platitudes. A well-spoken lady informed of my win. A cheque was on the way. I rang my husband, but he doubted me, and these were the days before scams. But this was fact, not fiction. I had won a prize. The cheque arrived! Our mortgage was cleared.

Later, I saw in our local Citizen paper a small random ad for a second-hand caravan in Wales.

I had no knowledge of the area but it called me.

Glynarthen, Llangrannog, Penbryn, £1,950. It spoke to me.

In a week, without a viewing, it was mine. I could not see it before eight weeks but it was my destiny. Family and friends had happy holidays. It was an ultimate experience. Sometimes, daydreams come true.

This could be useful advice, but only enter free competitions relating to mortgage advice.

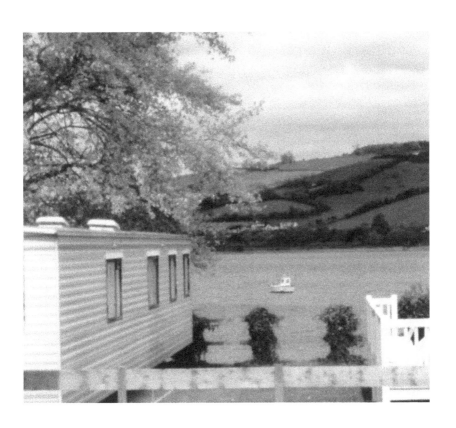

Alderney the Womble

Some people are remembered for inventions, discoveries, achievements involving a clever brain, hard work beyond compare. We revere their memory.

Better than nothing, my claim to fame still gives me pleasure.
The challenge.
A new Womble was about to appear on Wimbledon Common.
Find a name, the newspaper said.
My empty brain suddenly filled.
Why, surely, she would come from the same house as Elisabeth Beresford, the author of the books.
Alderney danced before me.
I wrote as I visualised her picking litter after a trip across the sea, then to Wimbledon.

Inspired by the jolly music of Mike Batt
Surprise surprise! I won the prize.
My husband, Mike; myself; young son David and his friend Matthew came too. In a first- class train, no less destination, London.
Met by a taxi, escorted on a trip of our great capital.
A weekend at the Hilton Hotel.

A trip round an animation studio.
Visiting a restaurant named Planet Hollywood, full
of stars. People, that is.
Back home.
Did it really happen? Yes, it did!
Thank you, Alderney.
My best friend forever.
I promise to always pick up my litter
on Wimbledon Common, as I did as
a child.

Now I read that there is a new book by Mike Batt,
"The Closest Thing to Crazy".

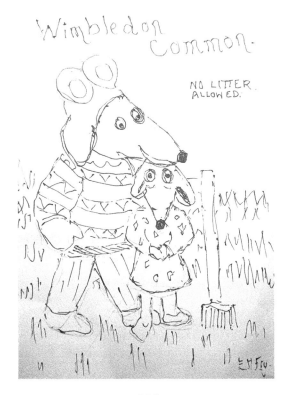

The Hidden Challenge

Many years ago, Robert Louis Stevenson wrote a well-loved book "Travels with a Donkey". He was exploring the Cévennes area in France, a magical vast forested terrain full of unexplored and mysterious pathways through vast forestland. To this day, very little has changed. Remote breathtaking beauty still beckons.

Sally's strapping son set out for a long trek and suddenly spotted, hidden in the undergrowth, a small dark back hole. It lured him in and, risking all, he struggled, wriggled and clawed his way inside. Inside and through a tiny gap, sweating and pushing and then panting, now too committed the hole to a cave growing larger and higher. He called out and his voice became a loud echo. Shouting in stock and amazement, he heard his own voice echoing. He wondered who or what had ever entered this place before. He was in a large and beautiful cave. He called out again.

Suddenly he was shocked by the confrontation of a large black bat swooping at him, prepared for a quarrel, and wanting to defend his territory.

Sally's son made a rapid retreat. He retraced his steps and struggled his route back to the light at the end of the tunnel. What an adventure!

Who knows what we may discover if we are brave and bold enough to take up a challenge and enter into that small hole of opportunity.

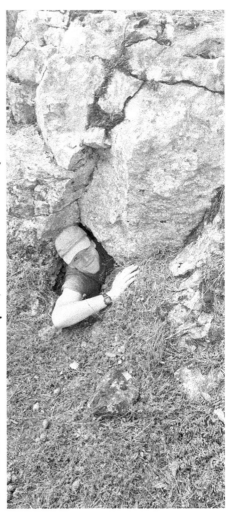

j'irai dans ce pays

117

Hurrah for Football

The game is finished.
No second chance.
Referee has blown the final whistle.
Ready or not, the match had to end.
Tense moments, crowds roared approval.
All was great.
Next minute, the opposition made their
mark with deadly accuracy.
The crowds shouting their advice was not
enough.
But
Friendships were made.
Players went the extra mile.
Tears of disappointment will dry.
There will be future opportunities.
Next time perhaps.
Bring it on!
No blame. No shame.
Just hope for the future.
Come on, England!

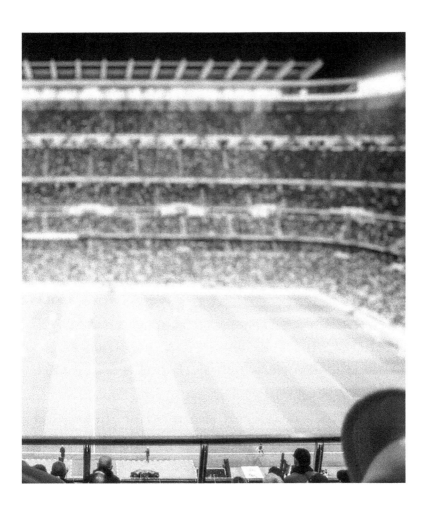

At the Foot of the Cross

'Why is he here?' the child asked, standing close to her mother.

'He must be a bad man, for that is how they punish bad people,' replied the mother.

A stranger next to them, forced to speak, whispered to them, 'He did no wrong.'

'Nothing wrong,' scoffed the woman. 'He must have done something. A thief, I expect.'

'Not a thief,' said the stranger.

'A murderer then.'

'Not a murderer. He always spoke of love.'

'Well, they don't hurt people for doing nothing,' said the woman, becoming bolder.

'Seems they do,' sighed the man. 'He healed the sick, spoke only of kindness, and owned nothing, nor ever wanted to. Last week, crowds welcomed him with palm trees and called him King.'

'Ah, King,' answered the mother, her child looking up at her. 'A King who loves everyone. No wonder they had to kill him. A man like that would change the world.'

The child searched their eyes but did not understand.

Eileen Fry

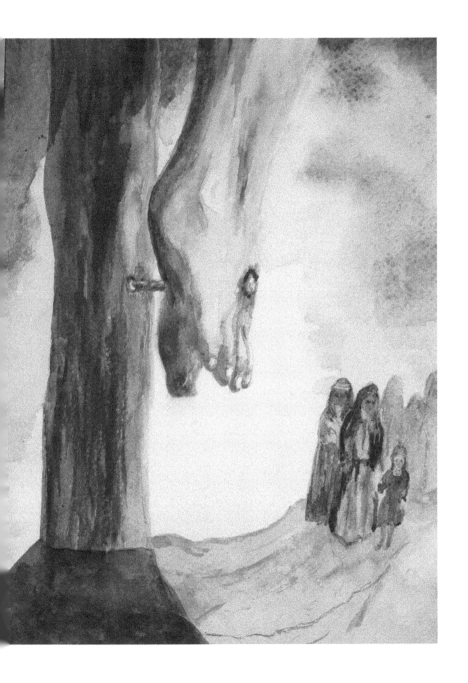